KAMA SUTRA

Master The Art Of Love Making Through Advanced Kama Sutra Orgasm Stimulating Sex Positions Guide, With Pictures

Table of Contents

Introduction

Congratulations on purchasing the book, **Kama Sutra: Master The Art Of Love Through Kama Sutra Sex Positions**. For centuries, the ancient Indian Hindi text of the Kama Sutra has been synonymous with discussions on sexual intercourse and the art of lovemaking. The full text in itself is quite lengthy and often tedious to read. In fact, Kama Sutra discusses more topics about human relationships beyond sexual intercourse, but it is the content revolving around human sexuality that has captured the attention of Kama Sutra enthusiasts for millennia.

Are you looking for techniques to enhance your sexual prowess, give more pleasure and satisfaction to your partner, or reinvigorate your sexual relationship or compatibility? In this book, you will find a concise, easy-to-read guide based on the texts of the Kama Sutra. You will learn techniques that have aroused the sex lives of couples over the centuries and gain a more thorough understanding of what Kama Sutra really teaches, apart from just the lovemaking secrets.

Don't delay your path to a more intimate, pleasurable and lasting sex life with your significant other. Start reading today and become the ultimate lover, ready to blow your partner's mind.

Chapter One: History And Philosophy Of Kama Sutra

For much of the Western world, the Kama Sutra is perceived to be mainly a sex guide. Although there are plenty of explicit sexual techniques presented in the Kama Sutra, only about 20% of the text actually discusses sexual techniques and positions. A bigger chunk of the text revolves around the path towards a life of virtue and grace as it relates to love, family, sex, relationships, and the human experience in general. Most of the Kama Sutra compares and contrasts various human desires, as well as the positive and negative effects of desire.

Scholars and historians maintain that the Kama Sutra was first written between 400 BC and 200 AD. The Kama Sutra in its current form was collated around 200 AD. The Indian philosopher Vatsyayana was the author of the Kama Sutra, and the writings themselves are part of a wider group of ancient Sanskrit writings called the Kama Shastra. Vatsyayana credits other Sanskrit writers' works as basis for his own Kama Sutra compilation, including those of Dattaka, Suvarnanabha, Ghotakamukha, Charayana and others.

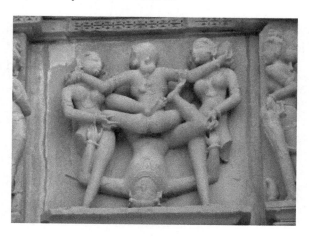

Image Credit: Shutterstock.com

The Kama Sutra text contains 1250 verses, divided into 36 chapters, and structured into seven general sections, namely: **General Remarks**, containing the goals and priorities of life, gaining knowledge and proper conduct; **Sexual Stimulation and Union**, with techniques on sexual stimulation, caressing, kissing, positions, oral sex and other sexual techniques; **Getting a Wife**, with instructions on courting a girl, different types of marriage, etc.; **The Responsibilities of the Wife**; **The Behavior of Other Wives or Concubines**; **Advice for Courtesans**; and **Using Occult Techniques for Better Sexual Attraction.**

In the Kama Sutra, Vatsyayana sought to highlight, or extol, the attainment of a virtuous life and how human desires are interconnected to this aim. The word Kama in Sanskrit means desire, and while this could pertain to sexual desire, the word may also refer to love, affection, wishes, or aesthetic or physical stimulation, not necessarily sexual in nature. Kama is one of the four main goals of life in ancient Indian philosophy, the rest of which are dharma (or virtue), artha (money and possessions), and moksha (freedom from the cycle of reincarnation).

The Kama Sutra teaches concepts on the pleasures of sensual living in general, based heavily on other Indian writings as compiled by Vatsyayana, himself a philosopher from northern India. For Vatsyayana, the study of sexual knowledge was a form of meditation, spirituality and oneness with deity. Although the text deals with many other topics, it is the sexual techniques of the Kama Sutra that have garnered the most mainstream attention.

According to the Kama Sutra, a marriage will be happier and more fulfilling if both the husband and the wife have gained a lot of knowledge and skills in the areas of physical and mental pleasures. The text consistently teaches that in the art of lovemaking, the mind and the body are intertwined, and for total intimacy and sexual compatibility to be achieved, both the mind and the body should be working closely together.

Much of the sexually explicit methods that have embodied most people's notions on the Kama Sutra are found in the second section, or the ten chapters dealing with sexual stimulation, desire, copulation, and acts. These chapters depict a wide range of sexual acts incorporating different techniques of kissing, biting, embracing, scratching, oral sex, intercourse, and foreplay.

The Kama Sutra is a notable work of literature in that it is unabashedly contrary to much of the Western mores and ideals regarding marriage and sexuality. While monogamy in committed relationships is extolled today, the Kama Sutra embodies the more liberated societal realities of ancient Indian Hindu philosophy. The Kama Sutra has an entire category dealing with the courtesan and how she can gratify her man, and chapters that discuss the relationship of the husband, the wife, and the concubines or other wives, a concept which is taboo in most Western cultures today.

Philosophies in the Kama Sutra often appear to be strikingly discordant, and yet somehow cohesive in their entirety. The Kama Sutra, for instance, has two chapters that deal mainly with the responsibilities and the benefits of the wife, while also discussing how the 'main wife' will deal with the concubines. The chapters on concubines and courtesans all somehow are covered extensively, but without diminishing the importance of the woman's pleasure. In particular, the Kama Sutra teaches that it is the man's responsibility to satisfy his wife's sexual desires, and if she does not gain this satisfaction from him, she may seek pleasure from someone else.

There have been numerous translations and compilations of the Kama Sutra texts through the ages. One of the most notable was the Ananga-Ranga, which was composed in the 15th century and is a revised version of Vatsyayana's original writings. However, because it was written in Sanskrit which is quite difficult to comprehend, translate faithfully, and study, the Kama Sutra became obscure for many centuries.

The Kama Sutra resurfaced in mainstream consciousness sometime in the late 19th century when Arabic translator and linguist Sir Richard Burton started on a translation of the Ananga-Ranga. Sir Burton's research into the Ananga-Ranga led him to unearth the original writings of Vatsyayana's Kama Sutra. Eventually, Sir Burton's work with Indian archaeologist Bhagwan Lal Indraji, Indian government officer Forster Fitzgerald Arbuthnot, and student Shivaram Parshuram Bhide led to the printing of an English translation of the Kama Sutra in 1883.

There have been various translations and revisions of the Kama Sutra in English; but to this day, Sir Burton's published version is still regarded as among the most accurate and faithful to the original text. Other noteworthy translations of the Kama Sutra include the work of Indra Sinha (1980), which contains the chapter on sexual acts many today associate with the text, and 1994's The Complete Kama Sutra by Alain Danielou. Danielou's work is noted for its use of original references to sex organs, and the use of original Sanskrit words in more contemporary contexts.

Is the Kama Sutra a guidebook for tantric sex? Tantric sex has a mixture of New Age and modern Western concepts interspersed with Buddhist and Hindu tantra and is nowadays synonymous with sexual practices and techniques that promote an elevated level of spirituality and sensual awareness. While there are some similarities and common concepts with tantric yoga, Kama Sutra is not a manual for tantric sex, contrary to many peoples' perception.

It is important to understand that the text of the Kama Sutra related to sexual activities are ultimately tied to its philosophy that human desires can be used to unleash a person's full potential, all with the goal of achieving virtuous living. The Kama Sutra does not contain practices or rituals that are tantric in nature, and it does not consider itself to be a sacred text for sexual rituals. In its philosophy, Kama Sutra is more humanistic, which sets it apart from the spirituality of tantric sexual practices.

Why has the Kama Sutra enamoured couples, lovers, and enthusiasts for generations? What are the advantages that this collection of ancient Sanskrit text can add to your sexual prowess or passion? In the next chapter, let us consider some of the appealing benefits that the Kama Sutra can offer to you and your partner as you ignite your bedroom activity and rekindle those passionate encounters.

Chapter Summary

- The Kama Sutra, although known primarily as a sex guide, revolves around the ancient Hindu philosophies of achieving life's goals through virtue.
- The original texts of the Kama Sutra were written between 400 BC to 200 AD. Much of the text we know today was compiled by Vatsyayana, an Indian philosopher and monk.
- The Kama Sutra is divided into seven sections and has 1250 verses grouped into 36 chapters.
- Only 20% of the Kama Sutra, just one section, discusses explicit sexual techniques. Other sections discuss proper conduct, reaching life's goals and priorities, types of marriage, rules for the wife, and instructions for concubines and courtesans, among other topics.
- The main tenet of the sexual lessons found in the Kama Sutra is the importance of knowledge and skills in the area of lovemaking, as a component to a happy marriage or partnership.
- In the Kama Sutra, it is the man or the husband's duty to provide sexual pleasure to his wife.
- Various English translations of the Kama Sutra have been published since the 19th century.
- Kama Sutra is different from tantric sex and should not be misconstrued as a manual for such.

Chapter Two: Benefits Of The Kama Sutra

It is interesting how the Kama Sutra has survived thousands of years and continues to be relevant and useful to modern-day readers. Even with the advent of technology and the many innovations and discoveries regarding human sexuality and interactions, there is something about the ancient texts of the Kama Sutra that still rings true to its followers today.

In many ways, the Kama Sutra was ahead of its time and is still quite bold and out-of-the-box in its views regarding sexuality and pleasure. Whereas much of the major religions and societal structures and mores have restricted open discussions on sexuality, relegating it to hushed dialogues or backroom whispers, the Kama Sutra fully embraced sexual pleasure as part of a healthy life. It promoted the idea that a person who is comfortable with himself or herself sexually, will also have a more balanced, well-rounded, and happy life.

The Kama Sutra also placed sexuality on a pedestal by teaching that sexual pleasure is a vital ingredient to married life. In stark contrast, many cultures and eras have often viewed sex as a necessary evil or only as a means for procreation and the continued propagation of the human race. Little regard was given to whether the man or woman's sexual appetites were being satisfied. In the Kama Sutra, however, sexual gratification for both partners is celebrated, studied, and fully explored in all its naked glory.

As is the case with any work of literature or prevailing school of thought, myths and misconceptions around the Kama Sutra have often blurred its essence, especially as it experienced a resurgence and caught a wider audience in the Western world. Many view the Kama Sutra as just a guide for different sex positions and techniques, or as a manual for teaching the man or the woman different styles of foreplay,

8

intercourse, and everything else in between. While the Kama Sutra does teach all of these, it goes beyond just the physical aspect of lovemaking. In fact, it treats lovemaking as an art, just like music, sculpture, or painting, with layers of intricacies and painstaking detail given to producing a masterpiece.

One of the biggest benefits of the Kama Sutra is its focus on bringing couples and partners closer to each other. Intimacy plays an important role in the celebration of sexuality in the context of the Kama Sutra, as it endeavors to make readers comfortable in their own skin. The Kama Sutra is an excellent way for couples to open up to each other and begin to communicate more seamlessly about their sexual urges, needs and sweet spots, all with the goal of satisfying one another.

Inevitably, as the Kama Sutra journey commences, partners become closer to each other as they also grow more aware of what the other person is thinking, feeling, and wanting. Sex, after all, can be a uniquely intimate expression of love and affection between two committed individuals, and the techniques depicted in the Kama Sutra help to further enhance the close relationship of two people wanting to satisfy each other in the bedroom. Learning the Kama Sutra techniques together means making discoveries, committing mistakes, and achieving new heights of ecstasy with your significant other, and this can solidify the bond that has already formed.

Another benefit of the Kama Sutra is its detailed teachings on oral sex. Fellatio and cunnilingus tips are dished out in the Kama Sutra and considered an intrinsic part of the art of lovemaking. While it is true that many people today are aware of oral sex and can perform it on their partner, many are unaware that there are strategies that can make the experience even more pleasurable, thus exciting and satisfying the other person beyond just the ordinary.

Also, considered a fringe benefit of learning the techniques given in the Kama Sutra, comes a boost of confidence and self-esteem for both partners in the relationship. When you realize that you are giving your spouse or partner wild orgasms or reaching the throes of sexual climax unlike ever before, this can elevate your confidence to higher levels as well. The Kama Sutra provides techniques on lasting longer and being able to make each lovemaking session more extended and packed with more action, so you can hone your skills and become that unforgettable lover you have always aspired to be.

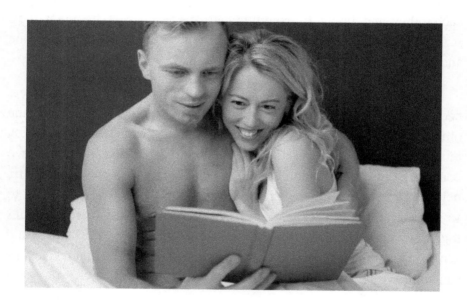

In relationships, the partner who is more attuned to the physical, emotional, and sexual needs of the other person increases his or her attractiveness. This is because you are able to reach those urges and cravings of the other person, and the fulfilment of these wants and needs becomes congruent to your attentiveness and ability to perform. Think about how memorable and sexually attractive you will become to your spouse or partner if you are the only one able to give them that intense sexual climax or mind-blowing foreplay they thought only existed in their wildest imagination? The Kama Sutra tenets increase your mutual attraction and will heat things up in the bedroom.

The Kama Sutra has a very positive, empowering, and healthy view of human sexuality, and it can help you or your partner overcome any negative perceptions, hang-ups, or experiences with sex. Many people are unable to fully enjoy their sexual appetite because of previous bad notions, misconceptions, or wrong expectations, and the Kama Sutra writings can help in correcting these misconstrued views and cultivate a healthier attitude towards this act.

As already mentioned, the Kama Sutra is far from just a sex guide that espouses emotionless intercourse between two individuals. Rather, it recognizes that the pleasures of sexual intimacy start in the minds and spirits of participants, so there are discussions in the ancient writings that deal with developing a closer relationship to each other. When the emotional connection is nurtured, conversations become more open and honest, and sexual compatibility also heightens. At the same time, when sexual gratification is fulfilled for both partners, the emotional and mental bonds are also fully engaged, improving the state of the relationship as a whole.

For the purposes of this book, however, we will focus mainly on the sexual aspects embodied in the writings of the Kama Sutra. In the next chapter, you will read about the foreplay techniques in the Kama Sutra, and its importance in the art of lovemaking. How do you heat things up in the bedroom through thorough, thoughtful and titillating foreplay skills? Read on to find out.

Chapter Summary

- Despite being written centuries ago the Kama Sutra is still as relevant to today's society.
- The writings of the Kama Sutra celebrate and embrace human sexuality as a healthy and normal part of life.
- More than just the sexual techniques, the Kama Sutra presents lovemaking as an art, not any different from music, painting, or sculpture.
- The Kama Sutra can help bring couples closer to each other, foster deeper conversations, and strengthen emotional connections.
- Successful application of the Kama Sutra techniques can elevate one's self-confidence as a lover and increase attractiveness.
- Oral sex techniques are discussed in detail in the Kama Sutra with the goal of pleasuring one's partner beyond their imagination.
- The ancient Kama Sutra texts promote a healthy and empowering view of human sexuality, thus helping to transform negative perceptions of sex.

Chapter Three: Foreplay Techniques In The Kama Sutra

Foreplay is the appetizer to the main course. Many couples rush through foreplay or even skip it altogether, getting to the main dish right away. However, extended and intense foreplay sessions tend to heighten sexual pleasure for both partners and can make the experience even more memorable for both. In the Kama Sutra, particular attention is given to foreplay techniques because it can set the stage for a more explosive climax.

Why is foreplay important? You can think of the human body like a car engine. When your car has been parked overnight, the engine has cooled down substantially and needs a couple of minutes to warm up in order to run better. During colder months, you may need up to ten minutes to warm up your car before hitting the road. You will notice the difference in performance between a car that has been properly warmed up against a car that is started and driven without ample time for the engine to get things warmed up inside.

In the same way, the human body performs better when it has been revved up substantially, and foreplay does this job. Men need to understand this part of the lovemaking process particularly because their female partner needs foreplay to really enjoy sex. Dr. Ruth Westheimer, a psychosexual therapist and professor/lecturer at New York University, Yale, and Princeton, notes, "It's particularly important for women to have successful foreplay because it takes a woman a longer time than a man to get up to the level of arousal needed to orgasm."

Men take a shorter time to become sexually aroused. In fact, a lot of men walk around with sex on their minds constantly and may only need a couple of minutes to be ready for action. Women, however, are wired differently and may need more attentive and thoughtful foreplay to be ready for sex. The female body needs not just the physical aspect, but also the emotional and mental preparation, and intense foreplay can open this portal in the female sexual experience more than any other aspect of lovemaking. Copious amounts of kissing, hugging, touching, caressing, and other foreplay induces the vagina to create lubrication, making sexual intercourse more comfortable and pleasurable.

Foreplay fulfills a dual purpose. It encourages blood flow to the penis, making it erect and ready for intercourse and makes the blood flow to the clitoris in much the same way as the penis. When blood flows to the clitoris, it becomes erect and more sensitive. An erect clitoris can be stimulated to achieve pleasure. Foreplay lubricates the vagina and hardens the clitoris, and this combination can make the sexual encounter more pleasurable for the woman.

Foreplay also gives the woman the emotional assurance she needs. The woman needs to be reminded that the man is not just having sex with her to satisfy his own needs, but because he genuinely cares for her and wants to spend time with her while being attentive to her sexual needs. When foreplay is extended, skillful and imaginative, it gives the woman the confidence that she has the full attention of her partner.

Kissing

For most couples, foreplay starts with kissing. Kissing can be done in certain types of techniques and positions on the lips and the body to create sexual tension. Specific zones of the body can turn on your partner quite significantly if you kiss the right area. Sensitive areas your partner will get turned on by are the Lips, Neck, Stomach and Inner thigh. Here are some of the main types of kissing as described in the Kama Sutra:

The Measured Kiss. This kiss refers to one partner offering their lips to be kissed but without moving them. The other partner will actively kiss the mouth while one remains passive.

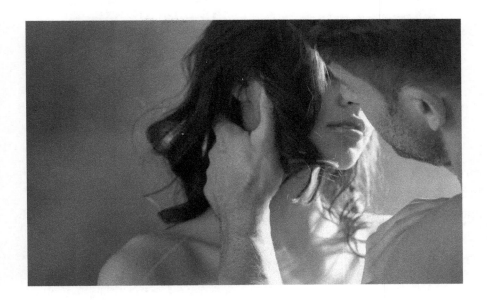

The Throbbing Kiss. In the throbbing kiss, the lips of both partners will touch, but only their lower lips will move. This may happen at the start of foreplay when the woman is still a bit shy and needs some prodding to release passion.

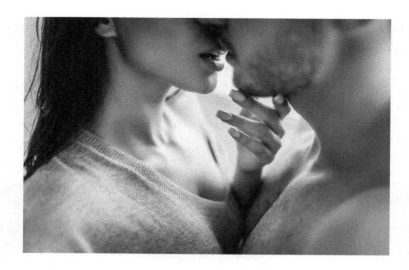

The Direct Kiss. As things heat up, excitement builds, and the direct kiss can be added. In this kiss, both partners face each other, press their mouths together, and begin to lick and suck each other's lips and mouths. Some biting may be incorporated.

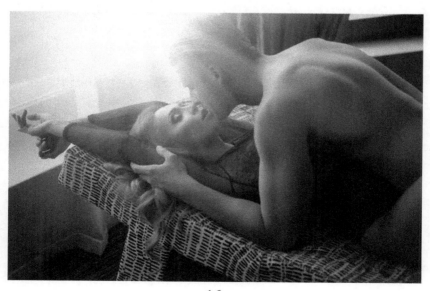

The Pressure Kiss. Couples who enjoy some aggressive foreplay can try the pressure kiss, where one partner keeps the other partner's mouth and lips closed while biting, kissing, and licking passionately. Holding their arms down against the bed or a wall will induce more sexual tension also

The Contact Kiss. In this kiss, one partner teases the other with a light, provocative kiss that only lightly touches the mouth. The partner then holds back while staring into the others eyes creating sexual tension from the get go.

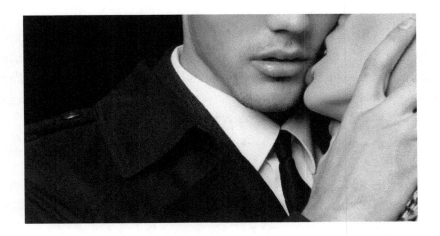

The Kiss To Ignite Flame. This kiss seems innocent but is designed to awaken the other partner's sexual mood. It is often used to determine if the other partner is still up for sexual activity. In this kiss, one partner innocently but seductively plants a kiss on the other partner's (passive) lips, usually while the partner is sleeping or resting, and waits for a response to determine if sexual activity will be welcomed.

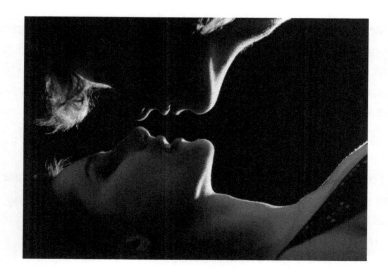

The Distraction Kiss. This kiss is not limited to the mouth. Rather, it can be used to warm up your partner by also directing attention to other parts of the body, such as the face, ears, chest, nape, neck, or shoulders. Many of these areas have very sensitive nerve endings and are called erogenous zones.

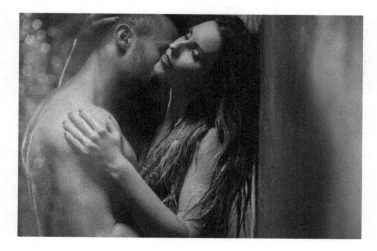

The Finger Kiss. A precursor to oral sex, this kiss involves putting one's finger in the other partner's mouth, with some movements inside, and then removing the finger and brushing it across the lips.

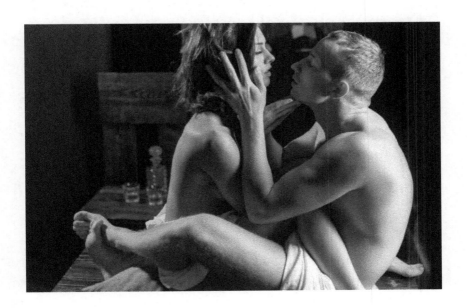

Touching And Body Massage

Aside from the intense and varied embraces and kisses in the Kama Sutra, attention is also given to other forms of body touching and massaging. Massaging can be especially relaxing and arousing to both the male and the female, and can be a loving, soothing precursor to the lovemaking session. In the Kama Sutra, these types of body massage are taught:

Face Down. This usually starts with a shoulder press, with the partner lying down on their stomach, while the other partner sits on their back and starts massaging the shoulders, loosening up the body and moving down.

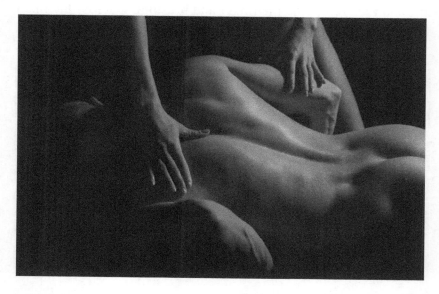

Rake Touch. As the body's muscles slowly relax and release tension, the fingers may now be moved lightly up and down the torso. This can be extremely sensual and sometimes quite ticklish for others. For added excitement, you may also use your lips or tongue to follow the same path that your fingers travel

Back Massage. The back massage must be done firmly but without digging into the body with the fingernails. The palms must slide and knead the skin and muscles both gently and firmly, with just the right amount of pressure. Strokes are done slowly and rhythmically, especially in the lower back and shoulders. For males, the lower back is an erogenous zone, while for females, the shoulders are particularly excitable. During the back massage, special attention should be given to the region between the buttocks and the spine known as the sacrum. This area is very sensitive to touch, and massaging this area with small, circular, rhythmic strokes down to the buttocks and thighs can heighten sexual arousal.

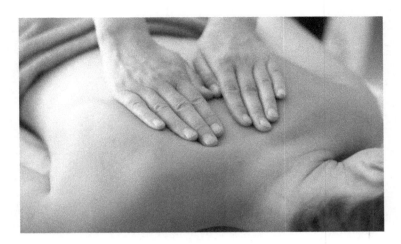

Thigh Massage. Keeping the hands well-lubricated, massage the upper and lower thighs with gentle kneading and stroking. This area is also very sensitive to touch, especially within the insides of the leg.

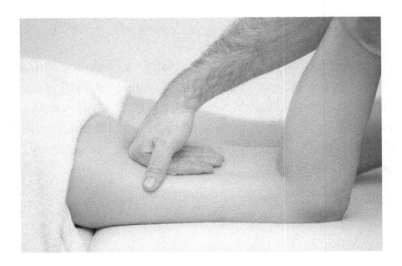

Release Points Massage. The neck, ears, and chest or breasts are erogenous zones for males and females. Small circular massages around these release points can arouse the partner.

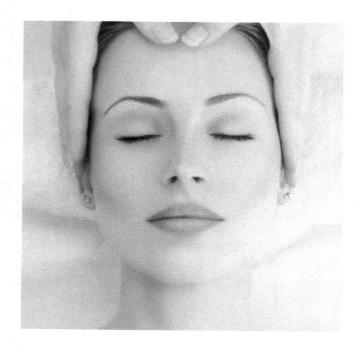

As you follow these Kama Sutra techniques on kissing, embracing, and touching, the sexual excitement will continue to increase. In the next chapter, you will read about the holy grail of female sexual organs – the clitoris. The Kama Sutra knows the intense power of this small but significant part of the female anatomy, and we will uncover its secrets.

Chapter Summary

- Think of lovemaking as a full-course meal, with foreplay as the appetizer.
- Long, thoughtful, pleasurable foreplay sessions add to the excitement of the lovemaking and build up the body to a more powerful climax.
- For females, foreplay is especially important because it induces vaginal lubrication and makes intercourse more pleasurable.
- In males, exquisite foreplay enhances the erection, while in females, it encourages the flow of blood to the clitoris.
- The Kama Sutra discusses several forms of kissing and embracing, all with varying degrees of passion and intensity, that are part of the foreplay.
- Foreplay is not limited to the bedroom. Throughout the day, couples may engage in foreplay and build up towards the grand finale in the evening.
- Body massage is also an integral part of Kama Sutra-style sex, with special attention given to sexual release points in the body.

Chapter Four: Clitoral Stimulation For Female Orgasms

As society has become more open to sexuality, women have also been encouraged to talk more about their sexual desires and needs. Men have always been quite vocal about their sexual gratification, but for most cultures women are not as frank in discussing what they like in bed. The sexual revolution of recent decades has opened the floodgates for more engaging conversations on the female body as it relates to sexual activity.

The clitoris as a female sexual organ has received a lot of mainstream attention, and yet continues to be shrouded in a lot of mystery. This female body part is still largely misunderstood by the male gender and often overlooked. Women, however, have become more aware of the promise of pleasure that can be delivered by the clitoris.

Situated at the top region of the female vulva, or external female genitalia, the clitoris has two main parts, namely the glans and the shaft. The glans is external and visible, about the size of a pearl, while the shaft is an internal part of the clitoris about one inch in length and running upwards from the glans. The clitoris has a piece of skin known as the clitoral hood which fully or partially hides it. Female natural secretions keep the hood lubricated over the clitoris.

The clitoris contains more nerve endings than any other part of the female anatomy. It is highly sensitive to touch or stimulation. When the female becomes sexually aroused, blood begins to flow to the clitoris, and it expands in size and becomes more erect, similar to the male penis (but substantially smaller). Clitoral stimulation is the surest way for the female to achieve orgasm or sexual climax, compared to vaginal penetration. In fact, the clitoris has no other function in the body other than sexual arousal. It is there precisely to enhance pleasure in the female, which is why it should be studied closely by any lover who wishes to cause toe-curling orgasms in their female partner.

You should note that the clitoris, being very sensitive, is a part of the body which some women would rather have indirectly stimulated than directly. The lips, tongue, fingers, hands, and penis may be used for clitoral stimulation. In the Kama Sutra, some techniques involve manual stimulation of the clitoris with the use of the fingers. You may start with one finger, then two fingers, with circular rubbing movements around the clitoris as the female adjusts to the sensation. Pressure and speed may be increased as the woman becomes more aroused.

During cunnilingus, or oral sex, the clitoris may also be directly or indirectly stimulated. The partner may lick or suck on the clitoris, stimulating the thousands of nerve endings in this body part, until the clitoris becomes fully erect. The clitoris may also be directly or indirectly stimulated during intercourse, as certain positions, such as the missionary, rubs against the pubic bone and indirectly, the clitoris. Whatever sexual position is being performed, either one of the partners may rub the clitoris during intercourse to heighten female pleasure.

Clitoris Stimulating Sex Positions

In the Kama Sutra, the following sexual positions are depicted as the most pleasurable for women specifically because of the clitoral stimulation involved:

The Mold. This position pertains to the man lying astride the woman and entering her from the side, which allows him to fondle her breasts, kiss her lips and face, and to rub the clitoris during penetration. This position is especially suitable for couples where the man is heavier, and the woman cannot support his weight. The angle also allows for deeper and more thorough penetration, intensifying the sensation for the man, while at the same time allowing him or the woman to access the clitoris or the breasts for female climax.

For women who like to have their neck, nape, ears, shoulders, or upper back kissed or licked during sex, the Mold position is particularly enticing. These erogenous zones are available to the man's mouth and tongue in this angle, and the man can send her to an explosive climax by stimulating her clitoris and nipples and kissing her neck while thrusting into her, all at the same time. The woman, on the other hand, can move her hands around his arms, head, or grip his buttocks during penetration, guiding the speed and depth.

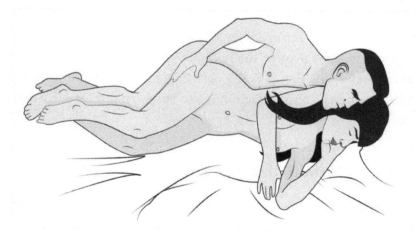

Face To Face. In this position, both partners are facing each other, with the female positioned on top of the man, and penetration is gentler but directly stimulates much of the front areas of the vagina, including the clitoris. As the thrusting increases in speed, so does the stimulation to the clitoris. Additionally, the man is free to caress or stimulate other areas of the woman's body. He can grip her buttocks, stroke her back, while she controls the speed and depth of the penetration.

Couples where the woman has a smaller vagina in relation to his penis would find this position suitable because she can control the depth of the penetration especially at the beginning of the intercourse. For women with smaller vaginas, the initial penetration needs to be done gently and slowly at first, allowing her organ to slowly expand and receive the penis. Because she is in control, she can relax her muscles and slowly guide him inside her, controlling the tempo until he is fully inside. As the intercourse ensues, the natural lubrication secreted from the vagina will make penetration more pleasurable for both partners.

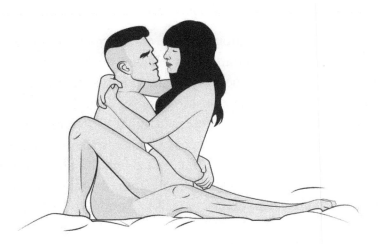

Missionary. This sexual position is arguably the most popular of all, and the easiest for both partners. At the same time, it involves a lot of friction in the pelvic regions and can be very pleasurable for females. In the classic missionary position, the woman lies on her back as the man gets on top of her, between her thighs, and commences penetration. During intercourse, the woman can focus on her pleasure,

27

and the clitoris is also accessible to both partners for manual stimulation. Women particularly enjoy this position because aside from the clitoral stimulation from the pelvis, there is face-to-face contact and a closer emotional connection to the man. Keep in mind that for females, sex is just as much an emotional as well as physical activity, and the sight of their partner on top of them, intertwined with their body, is a major turn-on for women.

Another advantage of the missionary position is it allows the couple to better angle the penetration, usually by adding a pillow underneath the woman's buttocks, to increase the stimulation of the clitoris during intercourse. This can be achieved without necessarily adding strain to either the man's or the woman's movements. Of course, as this happens, the friction intensifies, increasing the pleasure for the woman, while the man can thrust deeper into her nether regions, increasing the penile sensations as well.

The missionary position is one of the most intimate sexual positions in the Kama Sutra, and it remains to be among the most popular among couples, especially those in committed and long-term relationships. The missionary position allows for a lot of eye contact and is both physically pleasurable and highly affectionate. Kissing, caressing, light biting or spanking, and other sexual actuations may also be added to this position to increase sensations. Couples who enjoy a little bit of consensual domination or role-play may add blindfolding, tying, handcuffs, or ankle straps to the missionary position for variety.

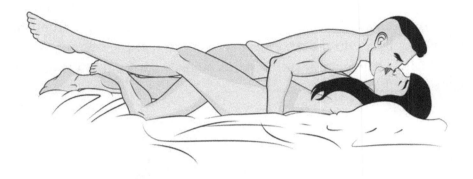

Delight. This position is often depicted in mainstream media and is among the most pleasurable for both males and females. The position refers to the woman sitting up and the man kneeling in between her thighs, embracing her around the back, while her legs straddle him. The angle of the penetration ensures constant clitoral stimulation, and the man is also free to stroke her breasts or kiss her upper body while penetrating the vagina. The Delight position is very erotic and sensual for couples. This position is particularly suitable for couples where the woman is too small to carry the weight of the man.

The delight position is also very intimate, like the missionary position, because it allows for a lot of eye-to-eye contact. As the bodies are more closely intertwined to each other, the emotional connection is also greater during intercourse. The woman can communicate to the man what other areas of her body she would like to be stimulated during this position, and he is free to kiss her ears, neck, nape, shoulders, and other areas of her upper body, while his hands can move around her back, buttocks, waist, hips, and other parts.

As mentioned in the earlier part of this chapter, the clitoris may be directly stimulated using the tongue, lips, or mouth aside from the hands or fingers. In the next chapter, we will discuss more of this in detail as we delve into the oral sex techniques put forth in the ancient texts of the Kama Sutra.

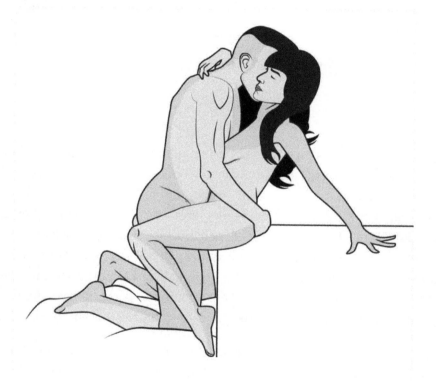

Chapter Summary

- The clitoris is found in the top area of the vulva, and consists of the glans (visible), the shaft (internal), and the clitoral hood (skin covering).
- The clitoris contains thousands of nerve endings and is the most sensitive part of the female body.
- Clitoral stimulation is the surest way to achieve female orgasm, more than vaginal penetration.
- The clitoris may be stimulated manually, during intercourse, or during cunnilingus.

Chapter Five: Oral Sex Techniques In The Kama Sutra

Oral sex may be part of the foreplay but may also be performed at any time during the lovemaking session of a couple. In fact, some couples may find it enjoyable to alternate between bouts of foreplay, penetration, oral sex, and other acts. There is no set rule that says oral sex should only be done before intercourse or as part of foreplay.

In the Kama Sutra, philosopher Vatsyayana discussed oral sex techniques in detail as part of continued experimentation and exploration of partners and couples. At the same time, Vatsyayana also wrote the text in the context of society at the time, where harems of the rulers had many kept women and oral sex was one of the methods used to avoid pregnancy.

Female Oral Techniques & Positions

Fellatio

Let us first look at some Kama Sutra techniques for fellatio, or oral sex performed on the male. Known in colloquial usage as a blowjob, fellatio is highly pleasurable for the man and can intensify sexual excitement.

Touching. This fellatio technique is described as the woman holding the penis in her hand, forming a letter 'O' with her lips, then touching them to the tip of the penis. Then, she moves her head in tiny circular motions. In this movement, her lips and tongue will focus pleasure on the glans or 'head' of the penis which is extremely sensitive, thus increasing his libido and preparing his erection for penetration. This technique is also called Nimitta and is a great first step for beginners who are giving fellatio for the first time.

During fellatio, the woman should be careful not to accidentally graze her teeth against the head or the sides of the penis as this can be painful. While some men do enjoy the sensation of light biting along the penis shaft, teeth grazing the penis especially during up and down movements can be painful. This is the reason for the 'O' shape which she forms with her lips, thus keeping the teeth behind the lips and away from his member.

Nominal Congress. In this oral sex technique, the woman holds the penis with one hand, places the penis between her lips, and then moves her mouth in a mild, gentle motion around the head of the penis. The nerve endings of the tip of the penis are very sensitive and this technique can be very sensual and ticklish. Again, the woman should be careful not to let her teeth graze the head of the penis. One technique that can be added to this fellatio style is licking the slit or the inside of the penis head. This area is very sensitive and can drive the man to near-orgasmic pleasure.

When performing this fellatio technique, the woman can think of how she eats a lollipop or ice popsicle. The movement is mild, a bit circular, and with the lips applying most of the pressure while the tongue is used to taste the penis as it is inside the mouth. Pay close attention to the tip of the glans and the sides of the head. The other hand not holding the penis may be used to stimulate the man's nipples or scrotum.

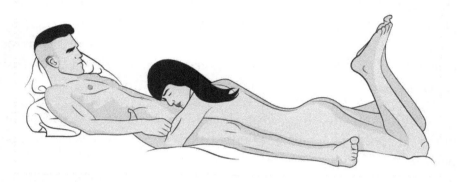

Parshvatoddashta. This technique is translated as biting the sides, where the partner grasps the head of the penis firmly, clamping her lips around the shaft, then moving from one side to the other, taking care not to bite into the penis with her teeth. The shaft will be gently caressed by her lips and tongue, creating an intense sensation for the male. The lips of the woman are particularly pleasurable to the man's penis because this closely resembles the vagina. In fact, many men find the mouth to be more pleasurable because it is more lubricated (due to the saliva), and because of the suction which can be performed by the partner giving fellatio. In this technique, the penis also probes the sides of the mouth, inside the cheeks, and the sensation can drive the man wild.

For women who have a gag reflex and find it difficult to take in more of the penis in their mouth, or if the man has a particularly large penis which is difficult to take in fully, this technique is suitable to try because it targets the sides rather than the inner mouth or throat of the woman.

Bahiha-samdansha. This fellatio technique pertains to taking the head of the penis between the lips, pressing it tenderly, and pulling at the soft skin under the head of the penis. This skin is very sensitive, so the woman should take care not to bite hard, only applying enough pressure to be able to pull the skin and play with it using her mouth. For men who are uncircumcised, many of the nerve endings connecting this area to the foreskin are extremely sensitive and can intensify sexual arousal by leaps and bounds.

This fellatio technique has the additional sensation of teasing the penis of the man in an area that is integral to sexual climax, but without necessarily moving the mouth in a way that will bring him closer to ejaculation. The teasing sensation can drive him wild and make the woman feel more dominant because she holds his sexual release in her hands, literally.

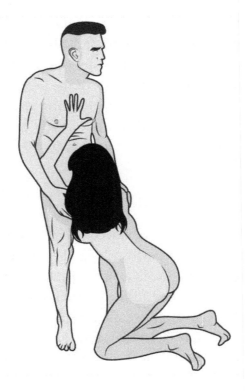

Antaha-samdansha. Similar to the technique above, this is also called the inner pincer. The woman lets the head of the penis slide fully into her mouth, then she presses the shaft of the penis with her lips, staying there for a few minutes before pulling away. The depth, pressure, and speed will increase as arousal intensifies. The man will feel his sexual excitement increasing as he gets close to the edge, only to be denied release as the woman presses the shaft of the penis, thus delaying his climax. As the climax is delayed, the penis becomes more erect and ready for vaginal penetration. The more rigid the penis when penetration ensues, the more pleasurable the sensations will be for the woman.

Chumbitaka. This pertains to kissing the penis as you would the mouth. The partner takes the penis in her hand, rounds her lips, then kisses the length of the penis while gently stroking. This technique explores the length of the penis, not just the head. As the woman's lips travel down the length of the shaft, she can use her lips to perform small sucking movements on the sides of the penis, while stroking the head or using her other hand to also lightly massage the scrotum. Many women are not aware that while much of the sensations are centered on the head of the penis, the shaft is also sensitive and needs attention during fellatio.

Parimrshtaka. This technique makes use of the woman's tongue, repeatedly flicking and striking the tip of the glans of the penis. Keep in mind that this is a very sensitive area, and some men may take a while to get used to the sensation. Other may find it too painful. The man must clearly communicate to the woman what is pleasurable for him in this technique and what he finds too painful. For most men, however, the tip of the glans can be stimulated with the tongue so long as it is done very gently and slowly at first, increasing in intensity as he gets used to the sensation. The slit is very sensitive especially when flicked with the tongue over and over.

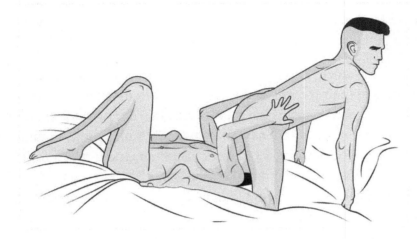

Sucking A Mango Fruit. Referred to in the Kama Sutra as Amrachushita, this technique refers to taking the penis deeply into the mouth, pulling and sucking vigorously as if sucking the mango seed. The sucking motion coupled with the sensation of the erect penis being fully enveloped by the mouth of the woman is extremely pleasurable to the man and can increase arousal, perhaps even bring the man close to a climax.

The woman can also use her free hands to stimulate other areas of the man's body, such as the nipples. The feeling of having the nipples stimulated lightly while receiving fellatio is very intense for the man. The woman can also roam her hands along the length of his body or use her fingers to play with his scrotum or the area between the scrotum and the anus. Many men also enjoy having their anus stimulated during fellatio, especially while the penis is being sucked deeply.

Sangara. This pertains to allowing the man to ejaculate into the mouth of the woman, using the lips and tongue to suck the penis until orgasm is achieved. The sensation will be very intense, and for many men the feeling of their intimate bodily fluid being taken in the mouth by their partner is an intimate and deeply personal act.

Some women, however, may not be comfortable taking the man's ejaculate into their mouth, so this should be discussed prior to oral sex. The man's semen contains the sperm cells, but also about 200 different types of proteins, vitamins, and minerals, including vitamin C, calcium, citric acid, fructose, lactic acid, magnesium, phosphorus, potassium, sodium, vitamin B12, and zinc. A teaspoon of semen, which is the normal amount excreted during ejaculation, contains between 5-25 calories, and the level of the compounds differs based on diet, exercise, age, weight, and other lifestyle choices. The fluid, then, is safe for the female partner to take in her mouth if she is comfortable doing so.

<u>Male Oral Techniques & Positions</u>

Cunnilingus

Known in modern terms as "giving head", cunnilingus is an act that the male partner must master because it can deliver massive waves of orgasm to the female. Here are some cunnilingus techniques taught in the Kama Sutra:

Quivering Kiss. In this technique, the partner pinches the vagina's labia, shaping them like the lips, and then gently kissing the area as you would the mouth. This is called the Adhara-sphuritam in the Kama Sutra. The technique is very sensual and intimate, and some women with more sensitive labia may find the pinching a bit uncomfortable at first. If this is the case, initial pinching should be done gently at first, allowing the woman to become more comfortable with the sensation.

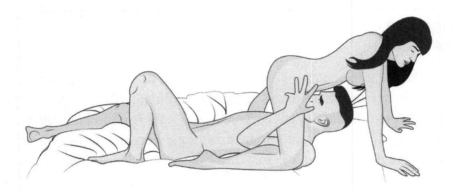

Circling Tongue. The Kama Sutra calls this Jihva-bhramanaka and refers to spreading the lips of the vagina and using the tongue to probe inside as the nose, lips, and chin perform a slow circular movement. The vagina is very sensitive, so this technique should be done gently. The man is advised to shave prior to cunnilingus to lessen the irritation that the female may experience when the vagina comes into direct contact with facial hair.

As the sensation becomes more intense and the man's tongue probes faster, the woman may want to hold the back of her partner's head and guide him towards areas where she experiences more pleasure. During this technique, the man may also use his free hand to circle her nipples, or caress her ears, neck, lips, shoulders, legs, and other erogenous zones.

Tongue Massage. This cunnilingus technique involves touching the archway of the vagina with the tongue, then penetrating slowly, increasing the speed and rhythm, until the vagina produces lubrication. This is called Jihva-mardita in the ancient writings. The tongue massage is great for foreplay and relaxing the vagina for penetration and is also a very intimate activity that allows the man to inhale and taste the nether regions of his partner.

As the tongue massage is being given to her vagina, he may also use his hands to roam around her body, stimulating her nipples, hips, legs, buttocks, and other areas. The female may want to arch her back a little and allow the man's tongue to probe deeper into her pleasure zones. For maximum pleasure, the man may also use one hand to stimulate her clitoris as his tongue is probing her vagina. Not only does this bring the woman to a mind-blowing climax, but the combined lubrication of his saliva and her vaginal secretions make penetration easier and more pleasurable for both.

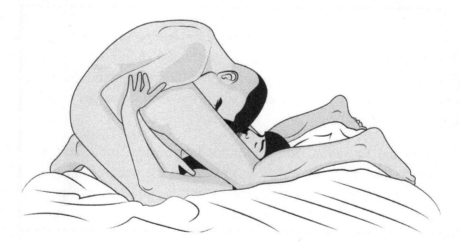

Sucking. Chushita, as it is called in the Kama Sutra, is the technique of fastening the lips to the vagina, then kissing deeply, nibbling, and sucking vigorously on the clitoris. As the man is kissing and sucking the clitoris and the outer areas of the vagina, he may also alternately probe the inner entryway of the vagina with his tongue or use his fingers to penetrate her vagina. This technique relaxes the vagina for penetration and is particularly. useful for women with smaller vaginas. As the vagina relaxes and expands, it also secretes lubrication, it will be ready to receive the penis, thus making penetration more pleasurable for both partners.

Sucking Up. Uchchushita in the Kama Sutra, this means cupping the woman's buttocks and lifting up, then using the tongue to probe the navel down to the vagina, staying mostly in the external regions. Circular licking and sucking motions in the area between the navel and vagina are very stimulating to the female. Additionally, some women find the sensation of the man's facial hair stimulating their navel, penis, and outer vagina to be very pleasurable. Other women may find this too irritating, however, and it must be communicated clearly. Irritation can be lessened through proper shaving of facial hair.

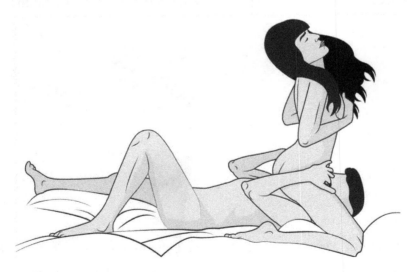

During uchchushita, the man may use his hands to travel around the woman's buttocks, occasionally moving up and down her back down to her thighs and legs. The woman, meanwhile, may use her hand to hold his nape and guide his mouth to areas where she feels the most sensations. The female can also move her pelvis in a rhythm to his sucking motions, focusing on her pleasure.

Stirring. In this style, the woman holds her thighs and spreads them apart as the partner uses his tongue to pleasure her inner thighs and vagina. The Kama Sutra calls this Kshobhaka. Adding the inner thighs to the stimulation of the vagina can be extremely pleasurable to the woman because the inner thighs are very sensitive erogenous zones. During stirring, the man may use his hands to travel the length of the woman's body or use his fingers to penetrate her vagina as he is pleasuring her inner thighs with his tongue.

For women who enjoy stimulation in or around the anus, this position opens up the anal area to the man's tongue, lips, and hands. The area just above the anus is especially pleasurable and becomes more accessible to the male partner as the woman holds her thighs.

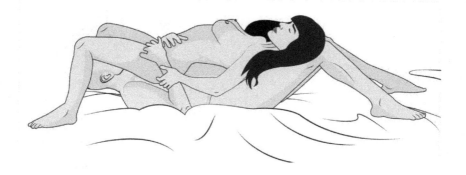

Sucking Hard. Called Bahuchushita in the ancient texts, this technique refers to setting the feet of the woman on the man's shoulders, clasping the hands around her waist, then sucking hard and long on her vaginal area as the tongue stirs inside. Couples who enjoy consensual domination or a little bit of role play will find this technique exciting, because the man now assumes the role of a slave who has no choice but to pleasure his female master with his oral skills. The weight of her feet on top of his shoulders may be moved closer to his neck, thus keeping his head in place and focusing on her pleasure.

In the bahuchushita position, the man's hands are on the woman's waist, where he is also free to move up and down the length of her torso. In this position, the woman's anus is also accessible to the man's tongue for stimulation, and if the woman particularly enjoys kissing in this area, she can let her partner know. The woman's hands, meanwhile, are free to stroke his hair, lift her leg up to make it easier for her partner or caress her own nipples and other erogenous zones as her feet keep his head around her nether regions.

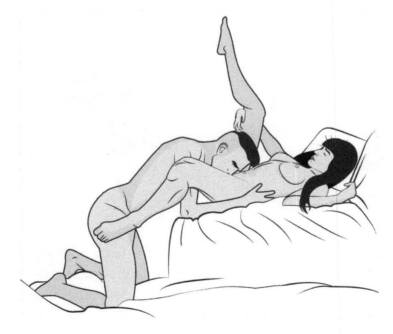

The Crow. In this cunnilingus technique, the couple lie side by side fronts toward each other, with one partners feet at the others'

head, while kissing each other's private parts. This is also known as the Kakila and is quite similar to the 69-sexual position. The Kakila is highly erotic and allows the couple to stimulate each other orally at the same time. Both the man and the woman are giving and receiving oral sex, focusing on each other's sexual sensations, while also receiving pleasure for themselves.

The kakila position is particularly helpful for couples who want to try the 69-position but may be constrained by larger weight differences between the couple. For instance, the man may be too heavy for the woman to have to support with her weight. In the crow position, however, because both partners are side by side, supporting their weight is not an issue. Also, the playing field becomes more equal as no partner has the upper hand. With both partners next to each other, all erogenous zones are accessible for oral pleasure.

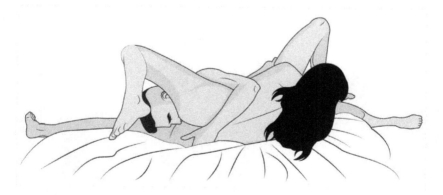

If weight or strength isn't a problem then the standard 69 position will be perfect because both partners get to enjoy the pleasure at the same time with their partners genitals deeply and perfectly inline for oral sex.

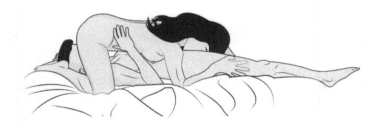

In oral sex, communication between the partners is very important. What is highly stimulating for one person may be uncomfortable for another individual. Some people have more sensitive endings in certain body parts than others, and this may require a gentler oral stimulation at first, building up to a crescendo of passion as the senses adjust.

As with any part of the Kama Sutra techniques, it is important that both partners are completely comfortable with themselves and each other, so letting your spouse or partner know what feels good and what does not is important. Instead of guessing or making your partner guess, be upfront and let them know what pushes your buttons. This is the goal of Kama Sutra, after all, which is to foster a more intimate relationship where both partners are attuned to each other's sexual desires and can give each other earth-shattering sexual climaxes because they already know what the other person needs.

After the oral sex practices given in the Kama Sutra, we now come to the sexual positions that the Kama Sutra is mostly known for today. In the next chapter, let us study some of the basic positions found in this ancient collection of texts.

Chapter Summary

- The Kama Sutra has many oral sex techniques designed for the mutual enjoyment and pleasure of sexual partners.
- Fellatio, or oral sex for the man, involves various styles that have varying degrees of pressure, speed, and motion.
- Cunnilingus, or oral sex for the woman, should be performed gently at first because the vagina is much more sensitive than the penis.
- Both partners are encouraged to clearly communicate what they like and do not like in oral sex. Some people's nether regions are more sensitive than others.
- Oral sex brings couples closer together and fosters a healthier, more intimately connected relationship.

Chapter Six: Beginner Sex Positions In The Kama Sutra

Aside from the Kama Sutra sex positions already discussed in the chapter on female clitoral stimulation, there are dozens of other sexual positions discussed in detail in the ancient writings. They range from the simplest and most basic to the downright adventurous. First, let us look at some of the more basic sexual positions as put forth in the Kama Sutra:

Blossoming. The Kama Sutra calls this the Utphallaka, and the position may remind someone of a cross between the popular missionary position and a Pilates bridge pose. In the blossoming position, the woman raises her vagina at a level over her head, and the man enters her missionary-style. This position is particularly helpful for couples where the woman has a smaller vagina relative to a larger penis for the man. The blossoming position is also a great workout for the female's core.

In the blossoming position, both the man and the woman see each other's bodies and facial expressions in full view, basking in each other's naked glory. The woman gets to enjoy her own pleasure while also taking in the sight of her partner thrusting and enjoying her nether region. The man, on the other hand, will enjoy the sight of her face revelling in pleasure, her body responding to his movements, and her breasts bouncing in rhythm to his thrusts. As such, although the utphallaka position is not as close in proximity between two lovers, it is highly erotic.

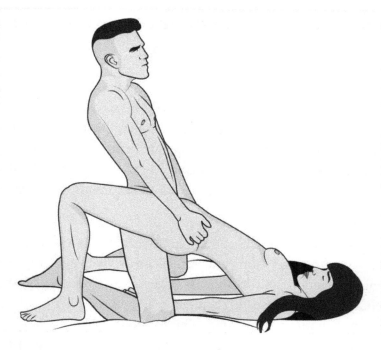

Envelopment. This position, also known as veshititaka, is particularly helpful for couples where the woman has a larger vagina and the man has a smaller penis. In envelopment, the woman will cross her legs as she is being penetrated, thus closing in around his member and allowing for more friction. Crossing the legs will make the entrance to the female vagina smaller, thus wrapping more tightly around the penis. During intercourse, the man will feel more pleasure because of the smaller orifice, while the woman's vaginal walls will also experience more friction.

In veshititaka, the woman may also practice clenching her muscles around the penis during penetration, which adds to the envelopment around his penis and increases the sensations for both partners. The position frees up the woman's hands to caress the man's buttocks or back, while the man can also stimulate her breasts, neck, or thighs.

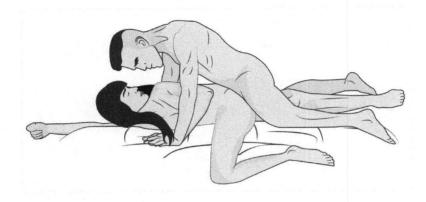

Expanding. This position is the opposite of envelopment. Called vijirimbhitaka in the Kama Sutra, expanding pertains to the woman raising one-leg during intercourse, similar to yoga leg lifts. The movement allows more of the penis to enter the vagina and is suggested to couples where the man has a larger member. In the expanding position, the woman lets the man fill her inner sanctum by opening more of her orifice to him. This position should be done gently at first, allowing the woman's member to adjust to the penis size, as the man slowly enters. More lubrication would be needed to make penetration easier especially if size is an issue.

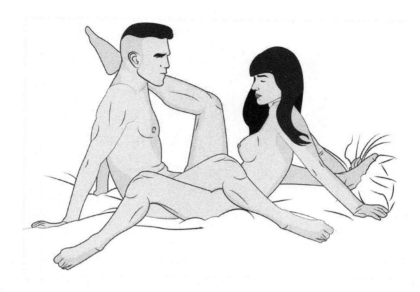

Impalement. Known in the Kama Sutra as shulachitaka, this position refers to the woman placing one foot on the man's head and submitting to penetration. It looks and sounds difficult but is quite easy to achieve especially for couples who are into erotic explorations.

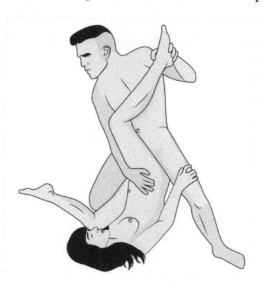

Lotus. This is akin to the lotus position in yoga, where the woman sits in a lotus position and then allows the man to enter her from the front. It does require some flexibility but is quite easy to achieve. The lotus position is great for couples who want to try sexual techniques that allow for face-to-face intercourse and lots of eye contact, but also need the increased penetration depth allowed by the lotus position.

The lotus position is ideal no matter the size difference between the man and the woman, as neither partner must worry about having to support the other person's weight. Both partners will have their hands free to stroke each other's hair, face, back, thighs, buttocks, and other areas. Also, in this technique the female's clitoris is easily accessible for manual stimulation, increasing female sensation.

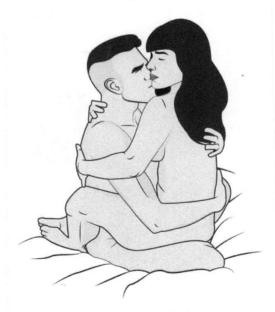

The Cow. In today's colloquial terms, this is now known as the doggy-style position. The cow, or dhenuka in the Kama Sutra, pertains to the man mounting the woman from behind as she is in mid-plank position. Many men consider this among the most pleasurable positions for them because of the angle of penetration. For the woman, the cow position also increases stimulation of the vagina because it allows for deeper penetration, and the man can also thrust in circular motions to increase the sensations. The woman may also reach under and caress her partner's scrotum during penetration.

This position is particularly popular because it allows either the man or the woman to stimulate the clitoris during penetration. As the speed and depth of the penetration increases, stimulation may be timed with the thrusts, inducing female climax. The man's hands can hold on to the woman's hair, shoulders, waist, or hips for deeper thrusts, or simply caress these erogenous zones for increased sensation. Many men also admit that they like the way their female partner looks from this angle, where the buttocks are in full view, the breasts hang low and bounce with the rhythm, and the woman's back moves with his thrusts.

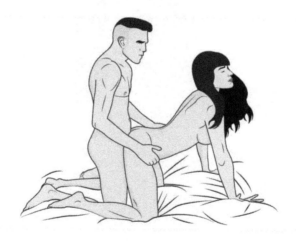

City Dweller. This position is big on eye-to-eye contact between the two partners. The woman will sit on the man's lap, facing him, wrapping her legs around his body, and then inserts the penis into her vagina. This very erotic and intimate position allows for a lot of caressing and clitoral stimulation. As the man penetrates the woman, he can use one hand to stimulate her clitoris, moving the other hand to cup her back or buttocks for deeper thrusts. In the city dweller position, the woman has control of the speed and intensity of the penetration, so she can focus on her pleasure and guide the man's penis into her nether region where she can feel the most stimulation.

The city dweller position is ideal for couples where the woman has a smaller vagina and wants penetration to be slower and gentler at first. To increase her arousal and ease the penetration, the man may also kiss or lick her ears, neck, nape, shoulders, or nipples, or they may engage in heavy kissing. As the vagina relaxes, more of the penis may be inserted, gradually until it is fully inside her member. She can then control the tempo until she reaches her climax.

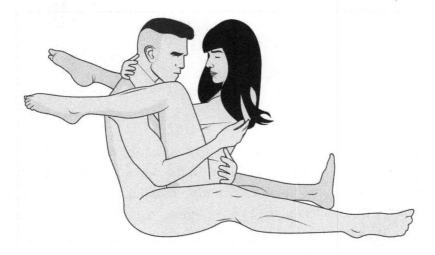

Lateral Box. This very simple sexual position involves the partners lying on their sides, facing each other, and their genitals touching each other. Slowly, the man inserts the penis into her vagina as they lie side by side, his hand guiding her closer to him. Kama Sutra calls this the parshva samputa. This position is great for partners who do not want their partner to have to support their weight, if they want to be able to kiss deeply during intercourse, or if either partner enjoys cupping the other person's buttocks during sex.

Many couples enjoy this position because it is not as physically strenuous. If you have both had a long day or just want to relax after a long time of travel but would still like to enjoy a hot bout of lovemaking, the lateral box is very laid-back and intimate. The tempo does not have to be rushed, and you can draw it out if you want, taking your time to enjoy the feeling of being connected physically while looking at each other and relishing the emotional bond.

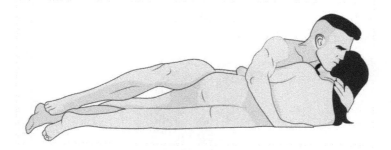

Closed Box. A variation of the style above, the closed box position or uttana samputa is done with the woman lying down, limbs stretched out, as the man is on top, pressing into her hips and penetrating from between the thighs. Again, just as the previous sexual position, the closed box is laid back and not as physically demanding, so it is great for partners who are feeling quite amorous at the end of a tiring day. Sexual intercourse can still be achieved but in a more relaxed and slow tempo.

One benefit of the closed box position is it allows the man to use his free hand to reach around and directly stimulate his partner's clitoris while he is penetrating from behind. Also, women who enjoy being kissed in the ears, nape, neck, or shoulders during sex will enjoy this position. The closed box leaves these erogenous zones free for the man to nibble on while he is inside her.

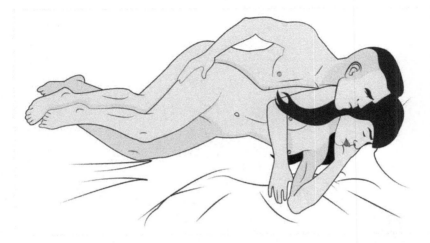

Frontal Box. Another variation of the box style is the frontal box. This time around, the woman has her knees folded up against her breasts as the man is penetrating from a doubled-up position in front of her. This position is suggested for men with large penises. In this variation, the form of the woman with her knees up against her breasts opens more of her orifice to his member. The angle will make it easier for a larger penis to then slowly penetrate, with the woman holding him and guiding the insertion.

In the frontal box position, the man also has access to the woman's lower back and buttocks, allowing him to caress or lightly spank these areas during penetration. Meanwhile, the woman can stroke his hair, face, or shoulders, or hold on to his torso as he penetrates. She can also reach inside and stimulate her clitoris as he is inside her vagina until she reaches her release.

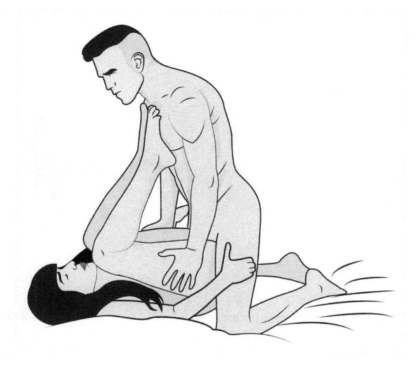

Bent. Called bhagnaka in the Kama Sutra, the bent position requires the woman to raise her thighs, her arms clasped over them and in locked position, as the man grips her and penetrates. Simple, but very sexually stimulating for both, this is one of the more popular of the basic Kama Sutra sex positions. In the bent position, a deeper penetration is achieved as the woman's pelvis is elevated, while the man's pelvic movements stimulate her clitoris. With the woman's arms clasped over her thighs, she can also hold on to his buttocks or torso during penetration.

Women who like deep penetration from their partner enjoy the bent position as it opens more of her orifice to his longer, deeper thrusts. At the same time, the man also has greater access to her clitoris and can stimulate it while penetrating her, increasing sensations for both. As the vagina secretes more lubrication, the penis slides in and out of the orifice with more ease.

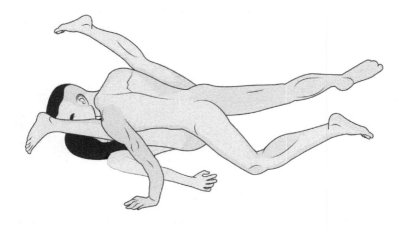

As you try these different Kama Sutra sex positions, remember to keep an open line of communication and ask your partner how he or she feels about each style. Humans are wired differently, and some biological and physical considerations and factors also have their effect on sexual stimulation and pleasure, so being open about what you both like and don't like will help you achieve that sexual nirvana together.

It would be helpful to have lubricating products handy during your lovemaking. Lubrication products such as petroleum jelly help make penetration easier for the woman especially for couples who contend with a smaller vagina size for her, or a larger penis size for him. Aside from lube products, sex toys such as dildos or vibrators of varying sizes may help her vagina relax before penetration, while also adding a bit of variety and imagination to the lovemaking session.

Now, are you ready to try some of the more adventurous positions as laid out in the Kama Sutra? In the next chapter, let us investigate the more acrobatic, challenging, and sexually-charged positions you and your lover may want to test tonight.

Chapter Summary

- Some of the basic sexual positions in the Kama Sutra mirror poses in yoga and Pilates, requiring basic flexibility and core strength.
- There are beginner sex positions for different considerations, such as penis and vagina sizes.
- In these poses, communication is important for the couple to maintain. What works for some couples may not be as pleasurable for others.

Chapter Seven: Advanced Kama Sutra Sex Positions

The sex life of couples can become quite monotonous and boring after a while if the same positions, activities, and styles are repeated over and over again. Thankfully, there are ways to spice things up in the bedroom and reinject life and passion into the relationship. The sections of the Kama Sutra detailing sexual techniques are particularly explicit about various positions that may appear to be more adventurous and challenging than the usual. These more advanced positions may be just the right ingredients needed to heat up your nights once again and rekindle that passion.

Before trying out any of the advanced Kama Sutra techniques, remember to keep the safety of yourself and your partner at the top of the considerations. Are you and your partner in generally healthy condition, and physically able to perform such actions? How safe is your environment? Are there potentially hazardous items such as furniture or lighting fixtures within the vicinity that may pose dangers if unintentionally toppled over or hit during lovemaking?

Of course, the comfort level of both parties should always be prioritized. Be sure to talk openly about what you both would like to try and set clear guidelines as to how far your sexual adventures would go. When parameters are set, stick to them and do not be afraid to voice out any concerns you may have about certain techniques you may not feel entirely comfortable trying.

The following are some of the more advanced sexual positions taught in the writings of the Kama Sutra:

Erotic V. For couples with that acrobatic flair, this is a must-try. The erotic V involves the woman sitting down on the edge of a table, with the man standing in front of her, bending his legs as he enters her. Then, the woman puts her arms back, leaning on the bed or table while wrapping her legs around his waist, as he then leans back and begins thrusting into her. Balance is the key in this position, so make sure you are both quite flexible (and the table is sturdy).

In the erotic V position, the woman is on top, but the man is in charge of the speed and depth of the penetration. She can cup his face, arms, torso, or buttocks during intercourse, while he can tilt her head using his hand, or grab her waist or buttocks for additional thrust. Kissing and necking are very much possible in this technique, and the angle allows for deeper penetration and greater stimulation for both the penis and the vagina.

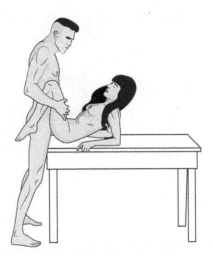

Fantastic Rocking Horse. For women who like to be on top, this position can be very pleasurable. The man will sit cross-legged and lean back, supported by his arms. The woman will then kneel over his lap, her thighs wrapped around his lower body, as she inserts the penis into her vagina. In this position, the woman has total control over the speed and the penetration. If the position is a bit difficult for the man to maintain his balance, the fantastic rocking horse can be done against a wall or bedpost.

For the woman, core strength and lower back stability are essential for maximum pleasure from this position. The fantastic rocking horse, meanwhile, is great exercise for the man's upper body and arms. Kissing, petting, and necking can be easily done in this position because the lovers are face-to-face. The man can stimulate the woman's clitoris as she guides the rhythmic movement, and use another hand to caress her nape, back, buttocks, or breasts. She, on the other hand, can use his shoulders to balance herself and help in the up-and-down movements.

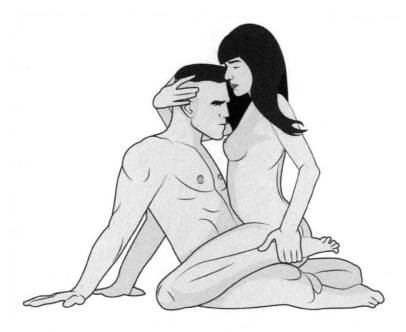

Catherine Wheel. Couples who are in excellent physical shape can try this position which is a bit more complicated than it looks. The partners sit opposite each other, face to face, then the woman wraps her legs around the man's torso. He penetrates her, wrapping one leg over the woman to keep her in position, while she braces with her hands. The man controls the movement using his torso, with his elbows supporting both their weight. It's a sexual position but can also feel like an upper body workout for the man.

This position has some similarities with the fantastic rocking horse, but differs with his leg keeping her in place, and with the man doing the movement. Couples where the man is larger in size and the woman is lighter or more petite will find this position very enjoyable. The vertical thrusting inside the vagina is particularly pleasurable for the male partner, while the woman can focus on her pleasure without worrying about supporting her own weight, or his. Their hands are also free to caress each other or stimulate the clitoris during penetration.

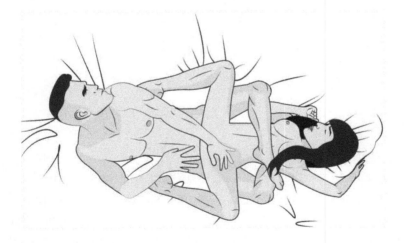

The Ape (Reverse Cowgirl) The Ape position is achieved with the man on his back. Then, the woman sits down, facing backwards, sliding his penis into her vagina as she keeps herself propped up on his legs. This very sensual position requires a lot of balance and coordination between the partners. If the woman is strong in the legs she can stand on her feet and squat into this position, controlling the movements while the male can rest so he has more energy for the next position.

Once this style is achieved, the unique angle will be intensely pleasurable for both partners. It is a different angle from many other positions in the bedroom and the male partner may find his manhood exploring new crevices in her special place he never thought existed. The woman will enjoy the stimulation in areas of her vagina not normally reached during intercourse.

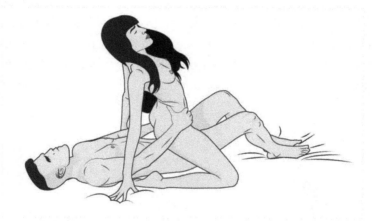

Ascent to Desire. For men who can lift their partner's weight easily, this position can be tried. The man stands with hips apart, knees bent slightly. He lifts the woman onto him, and as she wraps her legs around his hips, he enters her. In this position, the woman is in control of the penetration as the man supports her weight.

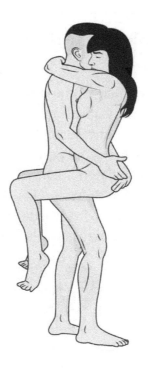

This position requires the man to be able to carry the woman's weight with his arms, back, and upper body. It is a great position for couples with bigger males and smaller females to try. The position allows for deeper vaginal penetration which increases the sensory excitement for both partners, while the clitoris of the female rubs against the male's pelvis and lower stomach, intensifying the pleasure. In ascent to desire, the man's hands may be solely holding on to her buttocks or thighs for support, but the woman is free to use her hands to roam his body. Kissing and necking are also ideal for this position.

The Bridge. This position is quite challenging and only suitable if the man is very flexible and strong. He will make a bridge with his body as the woman straddles him, lowering herself onto his penis while keeping her weight on her feet. The woman then proceeds to move up and down to control the thrusting. This position is great for couples where one or both partners have had some gymnastics or aerobics experience, or are active in yoga or Pilates, both of which deal with stability and flexibility and have poses very similar to the bridge.

In this style, the woman is completely in control of the speed, intensity, and depth of the vaginal penetration, while the man must support his weight with his arms, so no direct stimulation of the female clitoris or other body parts may be performed. The woman, however, is free to pleasure her own clitoris, breasts, or other erogenous zones while she is moving up and down on his penis. Couples should be careful not to do this position for very extended periods of time, as the blood flow to the man's head may get to be too much.

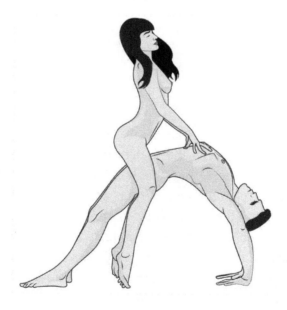

Double Decker. For small women and larger men, this position should be tried. With the man lying on his back, the woman sits on top of him, both facing the same direction. She leans back, propped up on her elbows, with her back against his chest. The man keeps her steady by holding her at the waist, penetrating at this angle.

The double decker sexual technique allows the woman to guide the man to those parts of her inner sanctum where she feels the most pleasure when penetrated. She can control the speed, angle, and depth, even moving back and forth or in circular motions to feel the full girth of his member in her nether region. The man, on the other hand, will particularly enjoy the vertical movement of her vagina on his manhood. The woman is free to also stimulate his scrotum with one hand while she is moving on top of him, while the man can use one hand to reach around and stimulate her clitoris and bring her to full sexual release.

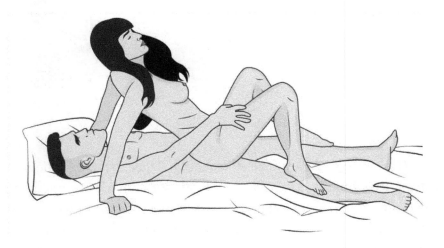

The Seduction. Women who have tried yoga may find this quite easy to master. She kneels and then leans back, with her ankles under her buttocks, then raises her arms above her head. The man kneels over her and penetrates from a planked position, keeping his weight on his forearms, thrusting into her deeply. In this technique, the woman opens more of her vagina to the man's penis, allowing him to probe deeper into every nook and cranny of her body. The arms raised over her head denotes complete surrender to his domination and the sexual pleasure that will follow.

In the seduction position, the man is free to control the speed, depth, and intensity of the penetration while looking into the eyes of his lover and watching her facial expressions as his manhood stimulates her inner sanctum. He may commence kissing, necking, or petting the woman while penetrating her, and she can also guide him deeper into her by occasionally grabbing his torso or buttocks and pulling him closer.

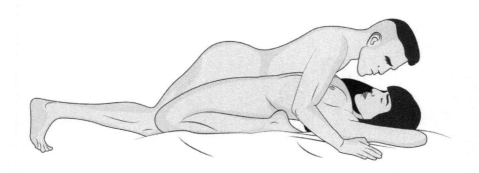

Crouching Tiger. The Crouching Tiger position allows the woman to stimulate her clitoris or his scrotum during penetration which makes this is an intensely pleasurable position to try. The man will lie back on the bed, his feet on the ground, and his hands holding up the woman's buttocks. The woman squats facing away from him, then lowers her vagina onto his penis. The woman controls the up and down movement while his hands help to support her weight.

This position has many similarities to the cow or doggy-style position, especially in the sensations as well as the angle of the penetration. The difference, however is the man is lying back in this technique, while the woman commences penetration by lowering herself into his manhood. Also, the woman takes charge of the rhythm and tempo of penetration in this intercourse technique. Couples who enjoy doing it doggy-style but would like to add a bit of variety to the position may try the crouching tiger. This sex position, aside from being very pleasurable for both partners, is a great leg and back workout for the female. It also allows the man to enjoy the naked glory of the woman from behind as he basks in the view of his partner taking him in and riding his member.

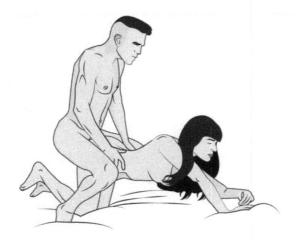

Broken Flute. This position is also called the venudaritaka and is among the most bizarre in the Kama Sutra. The woman lies down, puts her foot on the man's shoulder, then takes it off and puts the other foot on his other shoulder, all while he is inside her. It does require good core and leg strength, but the Broken Flute position is one you should try if you want something new.

In the broker flute technique, the movement of the woman's legs being alternately placed on the man's shoulders will cause her vagina to contract, expand, and caress his erection while inside her, causing an altogether different sensation. The movement also allows her to discover new areas of her vagina that need to be pleasured during penetration. The man will enjoy the sight of his partner taking in his erection and making it her own pleasure object, and during penetration the man can also freely roam the length of her body, even stimulating her clitoris which will be easily accessible in this position.

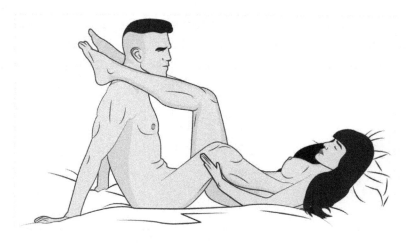

The Spin. In the Kama Sutra, this is the paravrittaka, where the woman is seated on top of the man during penetration, and then spins around 180 degrees. This is quite difficult for the woman to master but is intensely pleasurable for the man and the woman. The sensations felt in this circular motion are unlike any other sensations felt in other sexual positions, and there is also the rush of adrenaline due to the more physical nature of this technique, especially for the female.

Some women may find the spinning motion to be uncomfortable or cause a bit of nausea, so it is advised to go slowly at first, with the man providing as much support and balance as possible. The spin is one of the more adventurous and strenuous of the advanced Kama Sutra positions, but don't knock it before you have tried it. You just might find a different head rush when performing this position. For the man, be generous with kisses, caresses, and stimulation to her various erogenous zones before, during, and after the spin position to make the experience more pleasurable.

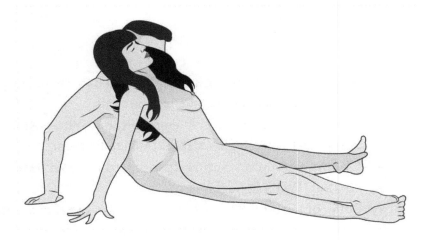

As you can see, many of these advanced sexual positions from the Kama Sutra will test your stamina, flexibility, balance, coordination, or all of these (among other skills). They may be hard to achieve at first, but once you master these positions, you will find your sex life to be more varied and adventurous. There are, of course, more positions detailed in the texts of the Kama Sutra which you can also explore as you become more of an expert in these styles.

Chapter Summary

- New and unique sex positions play a role in revitalizing a relationship that has become monotonous.
- Before trying the more challenging Kama Sutra positions, ensure that you are physically fit to handle them.
- Discuss with your partner first regarding your level of comfort. When in doubt, don't.
- Some of the advanced sexual positions in the Kama Sutra allow the woman to be on top and in control of the penetration depth and speed.
- For advanced sexual positions, the man must remember to also use his hands to stimulate the woman's clitoris, breasts, and other erogenous zones during penetration.

Final Words

Sex should be viewed as a healthy and normal part of your relationship with your partner. The level of intimacy and compatibility you reach with your significant other is undeniably tied to your sexual relationship. When there is conflict or unresolved tension, sex is often one of those activities that tends to fall by the wayside because it requires a level of closeness and emotional connection unlike any other activity. Likewise, a healthy relationship also often translates to an open and vibrant sex life.

It is true that sex is not all there is to a romantic relationship, but it cannot be denied that it does play a major part in the dynamics of the partnership. As human beings, our sexuality is part of who we are. It is wired into our thinking and plays a big role in much of our daily thinking and decision making, whether we are aware of it or not. Because of this fact, it is important to maintain a balanced, well-rounded view of sexuality in general if true happiness and satisfaction in life is to be achieved.

The beauty of the Kama Sutra is the unashamed way it ties together various sexual topics into its other lessons on life and the pursuit of happiness. That is why, even in this modern age, the tenets of the Kama Sutra continue to be used and studied by people all over the world looking to enhance their lovemaking prowess. While not necessarily an exclusive sex manual, the Kama Sutra has become known as the standard by which most other depictions of human sexuality and behavior are measured against.

How should these learnings affect you in a positive and enriching way? Hopefully, as you become familiar with the Kama Sutra through the pages of this book, you become more attuned to your sexual skills and the needs of your partner and develop a path towards achieving that peak of sexual pleasure together. Sexual intimacy is more than just an orgasm at the end of the act of lovemaking. Intimacy encompasses daily life and brings the couple together, allowing them to see the world differently and with the same perspective.

Through the ancient writings of the Kama Sutra, the hope is that you will enhance your skills as a lover, with the focus not on your personal gratification but on pleasuring your significant other, keeping his or her physical needs ahead of yours. The mastery of the techniques of the Kama Sutra should bring out that amazing and unforgettable lover in you. Through these techniques, you can reignite the fires of desire and connect with your partner sexually as if it were your first time all over again.

The Kama Sutra, with its valuable lessons on life, happiness, sexuality, and the human experience, continues to transcend generations and appeal to enthusiasts regardless of what era in human history they may come from. Hopefully, through the concepts of lovemaking portrayed in the Kama Sutra, you will begin to see sex as an art, requiring attention to detail and constant analysis of one's skills in order to produce a masterpiece.

By now you should have a huge understanding of Kama Sutra and the techniques & positions needed in order to reach the climax of your partner. If you found this book helpful please leave a positive review on Amazon as it is greatly appreciated and keeps me being able to deliver high quality books.

Lightning Source UK Ltd.
Milton Keynes UK
UKHW021546191220
375447UK00011B/2283